An
Se
Cu

Contents

Intention of this Guide 2

Passport Introduction 4

Let's Eat American Steak
& Seafood Cuisine 10

Let's Eat Mexican Cuisine 56

About the Authors and
Additional Products 102

Intention of this Guide

This guide—*American Steak & Seafood and Mexican Cuisine Passport,* is intended to provide information useful to people living with food allergies and specialized diets. AllergyFree Passport™, LLC as the authors, R & R Publishing, LLC as the publisher, the contributors and reviewers of this guide (collectively "we") have made reasonable efforts to make sure that the information provided is accurate and complete. We believe that factual information contained in this guide was correct to the best of our knowledge at the time of publication. However, we do not warrant or guarantee that any of the information is accurate or complete. It is not possible for us to have gathered all the information available or independently analyzed or tested the information.

We assume no responsibility for errors, inaccuracies, omissions or typographical errors contained in this guide. We expressly disclaim responsibility for any adverse effects arising from the use or application of the information contained herein, as well as responsibility for any liability, injury, loss or damage, whether it be actual, special, consequential, personal or otherwise, which is incurred or allegedly incurred as a direct or indirect consequence of the use and application of any of the contents of this guide or for references made within it.

The information contained in this guide should not be viewed as medical advice. Questions regarding specific food allergies, specialized diets, drug and food interactions and anything related to a specific individual should be addressed to a doctor or other medical practitioner.

We are not responsible for any goods and/or services referred to in this guide. By providing this information, we do not endorse any business or advocate the use of any products or services referred to in this guide, and the owners or operators of the businesses referred to in this guide do not endorse AllergyFree Passport™, LLC or R & R Publishing, LLC. We expressly disclaim any liability relating to the use of any goods and/or services referred to in this guide.

Although the authors and the publishers of this guide are appreciative of the support and information received, AllergyFree Passport™, LLC and R & R Publishing, LLC are not affiliated with (and have not received any compensation from or related to) any of the individuals, restaurants or businesses identified in this guide.

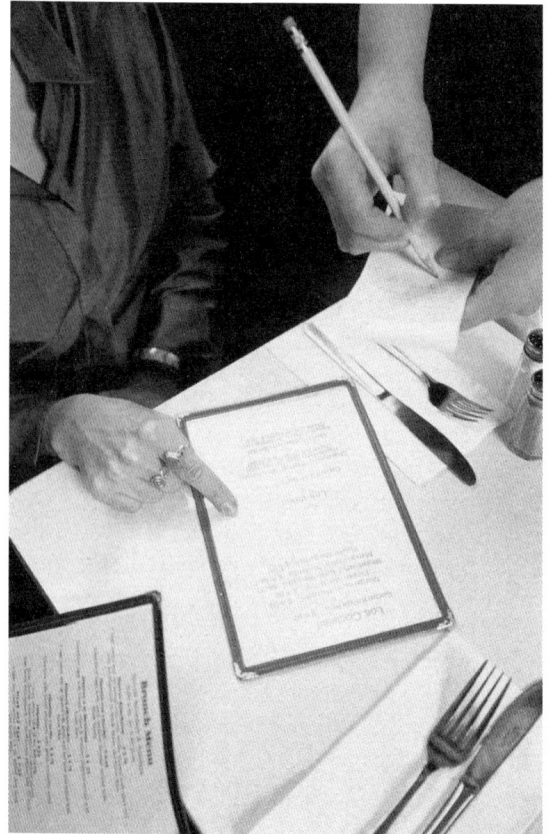

"If I have helped just one person in exploring a new location, be it in the city or country side, within their own country and/or on foreign lands, I will feel as though I have succeeded."
—Ralph Waldo Emerson

Passport Introduction

Overview

As part of the *Let's Eat Out!* Series, the *American Steak & Seafood and Mexican Cuisine Passport* is the first pocket reference guide dedicated to eating outside the home by respective cuisine while managing 10 common food allergens including: corn, dairy, eggs, fish, gluten, peanuts, shellfish, soy, tree nuts and wheat. This pioneering effort focuses on what you can eat by providing allergy considerations for 60-plus sample menu items from these two international cuisines. The contents of this passport are based on years of personal experience, extensive research, proven results and the collaborative efforts of many individuals and organizations around the world. This light-weight passport is designed to facilitate a safe eating experience whether you are traveling around the corner from your home or around the world.

Passport Approach

The passport is organized in a manner that allows you to use the information in a number of different ways. One of our key guiding principles was to develop an easy-to-use guide that is succinct and flexible to meet an individual's needs. It can be read cover to cover as a reference guide or if you prefer, you can skip around depending upon what cuisine or menu items you are most interested in learning about. For example, if you're planning to go to a restaurant, you may want to learn about the cuisine, potential menu items, associated guidelines and how to navigate through the restaurant menu. If you just need to re-familiarize yourself on possible choices or want a "cheat sheet" to bring with you to help guide your choices, you can view the *Quick Reference Guides*. It's all about your needs, preferences and areas of concern during that particular moment of the day.

Design and Methodology

The format is standardized across the cuisines, allowing you, the reader to easily recognize each section of information. The *Dining Considerations* outline how menus may be presented as well as relevant cultural customs and service styles for each cuisine. The *Sample Cuisine Menus* identify the name of each dish in its native language with the English equivalent. In our global research, we discovered that international cuisines often present each menu item in the language of the country you are in, as well as the native language. We researched cuisine menus and recipes from all over the world to determine which items are most commonly found in each cuisine. Once established, we reviewed each menu item to determine which dishes had the highest likelihood of being gluten/wheat-free. We further narrowed the selection by determining which menu items had the highest likelihood of not including the eight other common food allergens discussed in this passport.

Cuisine Menu Item Descriptions summarize each dish's ingredients and the culinary preparation techniques involved in its creation. We determined what areas of food preparation had to be confirmed with the restaurant to ensure each dish was gluten/wheat-free, what other common food allergens could be potentially included and the areas of food preparation that must be questioned to ensure an allergy-free dining experience. After each description, we outline the following concerns:

Gluten-Free Decision Factors:
- "Ensure" an ingredient is not present as part of the food preparation
- "Request" an item is not included or inquire about a substitution

Food Allergen Preparation Considerations:
- "Contains" an allergen from an ingredient in alphabetical order
- "May contain" an allergen from an ingredient in alphabetical order

The *Cuisine Quick Reference Guides* are designed to give you easy access to information discussed in the menu item descriptions. It provides an overview of each item in the sample menus and indicates whether a dish "typically contains" or "may contain" an allergen. These guides highlight what you need to be aware of to order applicable menu items, avoid specific allergens and adhere to your specialized diet at a glance.

About the Authors and Additional Products outlines background details and product information.

This passport can be used as a daily resource, a reference guide, an educational tool or a training manual depending upon your perspective. We hope it meets your diverse needs and empowers you with the knowledge to achieve your desired gluten and allergy-free objectives.

And remember,

> **"Life loves to be taken by
> the lapel and told,
> 'I am with you kid. Let's go!'"**
> – Maya Angelou

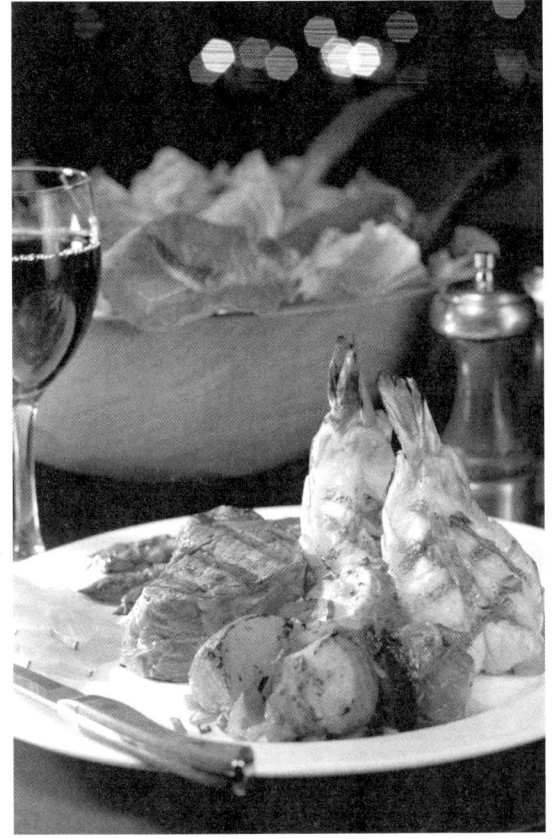

Of all the contributions this country has made to dining out, none is so quintessentially American as the Steak House.
—John Mariani

Let's Eat American Steak and Seafood

Cuisine Overview

The following materials outline:

- Dining considerations
- Sample American Steak & Seafood menu
- American Steak & Seafood cuisine menu items and descriptions
- Quick reference guide

Dining Considerations

American Steak and Seafood restaurants generally offer a limited number of menu items. They are presented in the English language, unless you are traveling abroad. A few large restaurant chains have locations in Europe, Central and South America and Asia. In those countries, you can expect to see menus translated into the native language.

Today, the standard American Steak and Seafood dining experience begins with appetizers and is followed by soup or salad, main course, and dessert. Since most American Steak and Seafood restaurants serve *à la carte,* it may be necessary to order side dishes of vegetables and starches with your entrees. The portions of these side dishes are usually quite large, so be sure to order appropriately and consider sharing them with the table. It is a rare occurrence, indeed, to leave without a full stomach. If you order too much food, you may want to leave with a doggie bag—a very American concept!

Enjoy Your Meal!

Sample American Steak and Seafood Menu

Appetizers
Oysters on the Half Shell
Shrimp Cocktail

Soups
Bisque (Cream Soup)

Salads
Buffalo Mozzarella and Tomato Salad
Chopped Salad
Cobb Salad
Hearts of Palm Salad
Mixed Green Salad

Meat Entrees
Hamburgers
Pork Chops
Lamb Chops
Steaks

Chicken Entrees
Grilled Chicken Breast
Roasted Chicken

Sample American Steak and Seafood Menu

Seafood Entrees
Crab
Fish Filet
Lobster

Side Dishes
Asparagus
Baked Potato
Broccoli
French Fried Potatoes
Green Beans
Hash Browns
Mashed Potatoes
Potatoes Lyonnaise
Spinach

Desserts
Chocolate Mousse
Crème Brulée (Baked Custard)
Flourless Chocolate Torte
Fresh Berries with Whipped Cream
Ice Cream
Sorbet

We would like to thank Tim Gannon, Founder and Executive Chef of Outback Steakhouse™ headquartered in Tampa, Florida and Domenica Catelli, Chef from domenica's way in Houston, Texas for their valuable contributions in reviewing the following menu items.

American Steak and Seafood Menu Item Descriptions

Appetizers
Oysters on the Half Shell

Oysters on the half shell can be served raw with lemon and a cocktail sauce made of tomato sauce, horseradish and lemon juice. They may also be baked or poached in fresh fish stock and topped with béarnaise or hollandaise sauce.

Gluten-Free Decision Factors:
- Ensure no wheat flour in sauce
- Ensure stocks and broths are made fresh and not from bouillon which may contain gluten

Food Allergen Preparation Considerations:
- Contains shellfish from oysters

- May contain corn from bouillon and corn syrup in cocktail sauce
- May contain dairy from béarnaise or hollandaise sauce
- May contain eggs from béarnaise or hollandaise sauce
- May contain fish from fish stock
- May contain soy from bouillon

Shrimp Cocktail

Shrimp cocktail is a common appetizer in many international cuisines. Most restaurants prepare and serve this appetizer in a similar fashion. Large shrimp are steamed or boiled in water or fish stock, shelled and chilled. The shrimp are served with a cocktail sauce (tomato sauce, horseradish and lemon juice), lemon wedges and sometimes an additional mayonnaise-based sauce.

Gluten-Free Decision Factors:
- Ensure stocks and broths are made fresh and not from bouillon which may contain gluten

Food Allergen Preparation Considerations:
- Contains shellfish from shrimp
- May contain corn from bouillon and corn syrup in cocktail sauce
- May contain eggs from mayonnaise-based sauce
- May contain fish from fish stock
- May contain soy from bouillon and mayonnaise-based sauce

Soups
Bisque (Cream Soup)
Bisque is a cream soup that usually features seafood, although vegetable bisques are also common. There are hundreds of recipes for this soup, but most call for standard ingredients. The base of the soup is butter, cream, some type of fresh stock or broth and wine. Onions, puréed tomatoes and potatoes are common vegetables and the soup can be seasoned with anything from sea salt to saffron. Vegetarian bisques may also include any type of ground nut. Bisques are usually garnished with parsley and sometimes may contain croutons.

Gluten-Free Decision Factors:

- Ensure no croutons
- Ensure no wheat flour as thickening agent
- Ensure stocks and broths are made fresh and not from bouillon which may contain gluten
- Ensure no imitation crabmeat or seafood which may contain gluten

Food Allergen Preparation Considerations:

- Contains dairy from butter and cream
- May contain corn from bouillon and imitation crabmeat
- May contain eggs from imitation crabmeat and croutons
- May contain fish as an ingredient, from imitation crabmeat and stock if ordered
- May contain peanuts in vegetable bisque
- May contain shellfish as an ingredient and from stock if ordered
- May contain soy from bouillon and imitation crabmeat

- May contain tree nuts in vegetable bisque

Salads
Buffalo Mozzarella and Tomato Salad

Buffalo mozzarella and tomato salad is an Italian classic that has secured a prominent place on American Steak and Seafood restaurant menus. Large slices of buffalo mozzarella are stacked with freshly cut beefsteak tomatoes. Large leafs of basil garnish this dish, which is dressed in olive oil and sometimes balsamic vinegar.

Gluten-Free Decision Factors:
- None

Food Allergen Preparation Considerations:
- Contains dairy from cheese
- May contain corn from vegetable oil
- May contains peanuts from vegetable oil
- May contain soy from vegetable oil

Chopped Salad

Think of a chopped salad as everything that is crunchy in a salad in bite sized pieces. Most chopped salads include bacon, green beans, onions and tomatoes. Some restaurants may include other crunchy vegetables, chopped nuts or add blue cheese for extra flavor. Salad dressings vary from restaurant to restaurant, but balsamic vinaigrette is typically available.

Gluten-Free Decision Factors:
- Ensure bacon bits are real—artificial bacon bits may contain gluten
- Request no croutons
- Request no blue cheese which may contain gluten
- Ensure salad dressings do not contain gluten

Food Allergen Preparation Considerations:
- May contain corn from artificial bacon bits, salad dressing and vegetable oil
- May contain dairy from cheese and salad dressing

- May contain eggs from croutons and mayonnaise-based dressing
- May contain fish from salad dressing
- May contain peanuts from vegetable oil
- May contain soy from artificial bacon bits, mayonnaise-based dressing and vegetable oil

Cobb Salad

This classic salad was invented in the late 1920's by Bob Cobb, manager of Hollywood's famous Brown Derby restaurant. Today, it is considered an American classic. Mixed greens, preferably Boston lettuce, endive and watercress, are topped with avocado, bacon, chicken breast, hard boiled eggs, tomatoes and Roquefort cheese. The traditional dressing is Dijon vinaigrette, consisting of Dijon mustard, olive oil, red wine vinegar, salt and pepper; however, other types of dressing may be available and balsamic vinaigrette can easily be substituted.

Gluten-Free Decision Factors:
- Ensure bacon bits are real—artificial bacon

bits may contain gluten

- Request no blue cheese which may contain gluten
- Ensure salad dressings do not contain gluten

Food Allergen Preparation Considerations:
- Contains dairy from cheese and possibly from salad dressing
- Contains eggs from hard-boiled eggs and possibly from mayonnaise-based dressing
- May contain corn from artificial bacon bits, salad dressing and vegetable oil
- May contain fish from salad dressing
- May contain peanuts from vegetable oil
- May contain soy from artificial bacon bits, mayonnaise-based dressing and vegetable oil

Hearts of Palm Salad

Hearts of palm are the center of the sable palmetto, a tough-barked palm tree that grows in Central and South America. They are an important export of Brazil and Costa Rica, ending up on some menus in American Steak and Seafood restaurants. This salad usually includes hearts of palm, hard boiled eggs, olives and tomatoes. It is simply dressed in olive oil and vinegar.

Gluten-Free Decision Factors:
- None

Food Allergen Preparation Considerations:
- May contain corn from vegetable oil
- May contain eggs from hard-boiled eggs
- May contain peanuts from vegetable oil
- May contain soy from vegetable oil

Mixed Green Salad

A mixed green salad may also be presented as the house salad. It is usually a combination of mixed greens, cucumber, onions and tomatoes. Some restaurants may add bacon bits, croutons, shredded cheese and the type of salad dressing may vary.

Gluten-Free Decision Factors:
- Ensure bacon bits are real—artificial bacon bits may contain gluten
- Request no croutons
- Ensure salad dressings do not contain gluten

Food Allergen Preparation Considerations:
- May contain corn from artificial bacon bits, salad dressing and vegetable oil
- May contain dairy from cheese and possibly from salad dressing
- May contain eggs from croutons and mayonnaise-based dressing
- May contain fish from salad dressing
- May contain peanuts from vegetable oil
- May contain soy from artificial bacon bits, mayonnaise-based dressing and vegetable oil

Meat Entrees
Hamburgers

Considered an American classic, the hamburger's invention has been claimed by numerous individuals in the later part of the 19th century. In actuality, the hamburger was invented by the hoards of Genghis Kahn hundreds of years before the United States was formed. Although there are many styles of hamburgers, most are made with ground meats including beef, chicken and pork. The most common is the beef hamburger, which is made of ground chuck or ground sirloin and either grilled or pan-fried. In upscale establishments you can find Kobe beef burgers, which are made from a special breed of cattle that is fed a diet of beer and corn. Some restaurants may add bread crumbs to the ground meat prior to cooking. Hamburgers are generally served on a bun with pickles, lettuce, onions and tomatoes, with French fried potatoes on the side. Ketchup, mustard and mayonnaise are usually offered as condiments.

Gluten-Free Decision Factors:
- Ensure no bread crumbs
- Ensure potatoes are not dusted with wheat

flour or seasonings that contain gluten

- Ensure oil used for frying is designated for potatoes only and is not used to fry other items that may be battered or dusted with wheat flour

- Request no bun—order gluten-free bun if available

Food Allergen Preparation Considerations:
- May contain corn from bread crumbs, bun, corn syrup in ketchup, seasonings and vegetable oil

- May contain dairy from bread crumbs, bun and seasonings

- May contain eggs from bread crumbs, bun and mayonnaise

- May contain peanuts from bread crumbs, bun, peanut oil and vegetable oil

- May contain soy from bread crumbs, bun, mayonnaise, seasonings and vegetable oil

- May contain tree nuts from bread crumbs and bun

Pork Chops

Pork chops come from the loin of the animal and there are many variations of the cut. They are generally broiled, grilled or roasted, and may be offered marinated or smoked in some restaurants. Pork chops can also be pan-fried in butter or oil. Accompaniments vary widely from restaurant to restaurant and can include fruit relish, sauerkraut and sauces.

Gluten-Free Decision Factors:
- Ensure pork is not dusted with wheat flour
- Ensure no soy sauce or wheat flour in marinade
- Ensure no wheat flour in sauce
- Ensure no wheat flour in accompaniments

Food Allergen Preparation Considerations:
- Food allergens may vary depending upon type of accompaniment
- May contain corn from vegetable oil
- May contain dairy from butter
- May contain peanuts from vegetable oil

- May contain soy from soy sauce in marinade and vegetable oil

Lamb Chops

The lamb chop, or whole rack of lamb where the chop is separated from, is widely considered the most flavorful cut of lamb. It is taken from the rib and has a good amount of marbling, which provides the rich flavor. The chops are usually browned on both sides in a frying pan with butter or olive oil, then roasted to perfection. They may also be marinated prior to cooking and served with a sauce. If the menu description states that the dish is herb encrusted, bread crumbs may be used. Lamb chops and rack of lamb are usually served with mint jelly on the side for dipping.

Gluten-Free Decision Factors:
- Ensure lamb is not dusted with wheat flour
- Ensure no bread crumbs
- Ensure no soy sauce or wheat flour in marinade
- Ensure no wheat flour in sauce

Food Allergen Preparation Considerations:
- May contain corn from bread crumbs and vegetable oil

- May contain dairy from bread crumbs and butter

- May contain eggs from bread crumbs

- May contain peanuts from bread crumbs and vegetable oil

- May contain soy from bread crumbs, soy sauce in marinade and vegetable oil

- May contain tree nuts from bread crumbs

Steaks

Steaks come in a variety of cuts, the most popular being filet mignon, New York strip, porterhouse and rib eye. Steaks are generally broiled or grilled and seasoned with salt and pepper. They may also be pan-fried in butter or oil. Some restaurants may marinate their steaks or serve them with a sauce, usually a béarnaise, hollandaise or a reduction.

Gluten-Free Decision Factors:
- Ensure beef is not dusted with wheat flour
- Ensure no soy sauce or wheat flour in marinade
- Ensure no wheat flour in sauce

Food Allergen Preparation Considerations:
- May contain corn from vegetable oil
- May contain dairy from butter, béarnaise or hollandaise sauce
- May contain eggs from béarnaise or hollandaise sauce
- May contain peanuts from vegetable oil
- May contain soy from soy sauce in marinade and vegetable oil

Chicken Entrees
Grilled Chicken Breast

Grilled chicken breast is a relatively common menu item in American Steak and Seafood restaurants. In addition to grilled, chicken breasts may also be pan-fried in butter or oil. Occasionally, they may be marinated and come with a sauce. Fortunately, you can usually order a plain grilled chicken breast without any sauce. This entrée is typically accompanied by one or two side vegetables, even though many restaurants serve *à la carte*.

Gluten-Free Decision Factors:
- Ensure chicken is not dusted with wheat flour
- Ensure no soy sauce or wheat flour in marinade
- Ensure no wheat flour in sauce

Food Allergen Preparation Considerations:
- Food allergens may vary depending upon type of accompaniment
- May contain corn from vegetable oil
- May contain dairy from butter
- May contain peanuts from vegetable oil
- May contain soy from soy sauce in marinade and vegetable oil

Roasted Chicken

Chicken is typically roasted on a spit or in a pan with butter or oil. The chicken may be buttered, rubbed with herbs and oil or marinated prior to cooking. A reduction sauce may also be served in some restaurants. The common portion served is half a chicken, complete with breast, wing and thigh on the bone. This entrée is typically accompanied by one or two side vegetables, even though many restaurants serve *à la carte*.

Gluten-Free Decision Factors:
- Ensure chicken is not dusted with wheat flour
- Ensure no soy sauce or wheat flour in marinade
- Ensure no wheat flour in sauce

Food Allergen Preparation Considerations:
- Food allergens may vary depending upon type of accompaniment
- May contain corn from vegetable oil
- May contain dairy from butter
- May contain peanuts from vegetable oil

- May contain soy from soy sauce in marinade and vegetable oil

Seafood Entrees
Crab

Alaskan king crab, Maryland blue crab, snow crab and stone crab are the most common varieties of this crustacean offered. Crabs are usually baked or boiled in water or fish stock. The smaller crabs, like Maryland blue crab and stone crab, may be stuffed prior to baking and may contain bread crumbs. Crabs are usually served with drawn butter (melted butter and vegetable oil) and lemon wedges. Unless you are dining at the source of the catch, you may find that your crab has been frozen prior to preparation.

Gluten-Free Decision Factors:
- Ensure no bread crumbs if baked
- Ensure stocks and broths are made fresh and not from bouillon which may contain gluten

Food Allergen Preparation Considerations:
- Contains shellfish from crab

- May contain corn from bouillon, bread crumbs and vegetable oil in drawn butter

- May contain dairy from bread crumbs and drawn butter

- May contain eggs from bread crumbs

- May contain fish from fish stock

- May contain peanuts from bread crumbs and vegetable oil

- May contain soy from bouillon, bread crumbs, and vegetable oil in drawn butter

- May contain tree nuts from bread crumbs

Fish Filet

Most restaurants offer a fish of the day, which usually revolves around what is in season. Halibut, salmon and sea bass are very common, with many restaurants also offering fresh water fish such as rainbow trout. Fish filets are usually grilled, poached or steamed. They may also be pan-fried with butter or oil and topped with a number of different sauces.

Gluten-Free Decision Factors:
- Ensure no wheat flour in sauce
- Ensure stocks and broths are made fresh and not from bouillon which may contain gluten if poached

Food Allergen Preparation Considerations:
- Contains fish
- May contain corn from bouillon and vegetable oil
- May contain dairy from butter
- May contain peanuts from vegetable oil
- May contain soy from bouillon and vegetable oil

Lobster

There are two types of lobster typically served at American Steak and Seafood restaurants: Australian and Maine. Australian lobster is known for its large flavorful tail and is usually frozen prior to preparation. Maine lobsters are widely considered to have the sweetest flavor and are typically fresh or live prior to cooking. Lobster tails are usually baked or grilled; whereas, whole Maine lobster is traditionally boiled in water or fish stock. Most lobster is generally served with drawn butter and lemon wedges. Baked Maine Lobster is often halved and topped with bread crumbs and fresh herbs.

Gluten-Free Decision Factors:
- Ensure no bread crumbs if baked
- Ensure stocks and broths are made fresh and not from bouillon which may contain gluten

Food Allergen Preparation Considerations:
- Contains shellfish from lobster
- May contain corn from bouillon, bread crumbs and vegetable oil in drawn butter
- May contain dairy from bread crumbs and drawn butter
- May contain eggs from bread crumbs
- May contain fish from fish stock
- May contain peanuts from bread crumbs and vegetable oil

- May contain soy from bouillon, bread crumbs, and vegetable oil in drawn butter
- May contain tree nuts from bread crumbs

Side Dishes
Asparagus
Asparagus is usually prepared in the French style, steamed until they are cooked and still crisp. They are often sautéed in butter or oil, with garlic or onions sometimes added. Some restaurants offer béarnaise or hollandaise sauce on top or on the side for dipping.

Gluten-Free Decision Factors:
- Ensure no wheat flour in sauce

Food Allergen Preparation Considerations:
- May contain corn from vegetable oil
- May contain dairy from butter, béarnaise and hollandaise sauce
- May contain eggs from béarnaise and hollandaise sauce
- May contain peanuts from vegetable oil

- May contain soy from vegetable oil

Baked Potato

A baked potato is typically a safe choice in any restaurant. The accompaniments vary from restaurant to restaurant, but can include bacon bits, butter, cheese, chives and sour cream. Cheese sauce may also be offered. Mix and match what you like or have it plain. Almost all baked potatoes are made to order.

Gluten-Free Decision Factors:
- Ensure bacon bits are real—artificial bacon bits may contain gluten
- Ensure no wheat flour in cheese sauce

Food Allergen Preparation Considerations:
- May contain corn from artificial bacon bits and cheese sauce
- May contain dairy from butter, cheese and sour cream
- May contain soy from artificial bacon bits and cheese sauce

Broccoli

In most cases, broccoli is steamed at American Steak and Seafood restaurants. You may also request it sautéed with butter or olive oil and garlic. In some establishments, the option of cheese sauce may also be available.

Gluten-Free Decision Factors:
- Ensure no wheat flour in cheese sauce

Food Allergen Preparation Considerations:
- May contain corn from cheese sauce and vegetable oil
- May contain dairy from butter and cheese sauce
- May contain peanuts in vegetable oil
- May contain soy from cheese sauce and vegetable oil

French Fried Potatoes

French fried potatoes come in many different shapes and sizes. Once cut, the potatoes are fried in oil. Some restaurants may season their fries, while others prefer salting. Ketchup is usually served on the side.

Gluten-Free Decision Factors:
- Ensure potatoes are not dusted with wheat flour or seasonings that contain gluten
- Ensure oil used for frying is designated for potatoes only and is not used to fry other items that may be battered or dusted with wheat flour

Food Allergen Preparation Considerations:
- May contain corn from corn syrup in ketchup, seasonings and vegetable oil
- May contain dairy from seasonings
- May contain peanuts from peanut oil and vegetable oil
- May contain soy from ketchup, seasonings and vegetable oil

Green Beans

Green beans are usually served in the French style, steamed until they are cooked and still crisp. They are typically served plain or sautéed in butter or oil. Other ingredients such as almonds, garlic and onions may also be included. Green beans may be served with béarnaise or hollandaise sauce on the side.

Gluten-Free Decision Factors:
- Ensure no wheat flour in sauce

Food Allergen Preparation Considerations:
- May contain corn from vegetable oil
- May contain dairy from butter, béarnaise and hollandaise sauce
- May contain eggs from béarnaise and hollandaise sauce
- May contain peanuts from vegetable oil
- May contain soy from vegetable oil
- May contain tree nuts from almonds

Hash Browns
Hash browns are a classic side dish. Julienned potatoes are simply pan fried with butter or vegetable oil, very much like a pancake. They are

fried on one side and then carefully flipped over to brown on the other side. Occasionally, they may have sliced onions added to them. Hash browns are usually only seasoned with salt and pepper.

Gluten-Free Decision Factors:
- Ensure no wheat flour or seasonings that contain gluten

Food Allergen Preparation Considerations:
- May contain corn from seasonings and vegetable oil
- May contain dairy from butter and seasonings
- May contain peanuts from vegetable oil
- May contain soy from seasonings and vegetable oil

Mashed Potatoes

Mashed Potatoes are made a variety of ways, most of which include butter and milk to add a creamy texture. The potatoes can be mashed, smashed or whipped with or without the skins left on the spud. Chives and onions are often added to the mix, with garlic mashed potatoes and parmesan cheese mashed potatoes growing in popularity. Salt and pepper are the standard seasonings used; however, some chefs may add fresh herbs to enhance the flavor.

Gluten-Free Decision Factors:
- Ensure no wheat flour as ingredient
- Ensure no artificial mashed potato mix which may contain gluten

Food Allergen Preparation Considerations:
- May contain corn from artificial mashed potato mix
- May contain dairy from artificial mashed potato mix, butter, cheese and milk
- May contain soy from artificial mashed potato mix

Potatoes Lyonnaise
Potatoes Lyonnaise are a French potato side dish, very similar to American hash browns. Potatoes are sliced or cubed and then pan fried with sliced

onions, butter, salt and pepper. Some restaurants may choose to bake this dish or substitute vegetable oil for butter.

Gluten-Free Decision Factors:
- Ensure no wheat flour as ingredient

Food Allergen Preparation Considerations:
- May contain corn from vegetable oil
- May contain dairy from butter
- May contain peanuts from vegetable oil
- May contain soy from vegetable oil

Spinach

Spinach is full of vitamins and makes a great side dish. It is typically steamed or sautéed in olive oil with garlic or onions. Creamed spinach is also usually available; however, most recipes indicate wheat flour as an ingredient.

Gluten-Free Decision Factors:
- Ensure no wheat flour in creamed spinach

Food Allergen Preparation Considerations:
- May contain corn from vegetable oil
- May contain dairy from butter and cream
- May contain peanuts from vegetable oil
- May contain soy from vegetable oil

Desserts
Chocolate Mousse
Chocolate mousse has become a popular dessert and can be found on the menus of many international cuisines. There are a number of variations, but the preparation is typically consistent with the following recipe. Chocolate is melted in a double-boiler with milk and sugar. Whipped eggs are then carefully folded into the chocolate sauce after it has cooled. Next, whipped heavy cream is added to the mixture, which is allowed to sit for a few minutes before the mousse is poured into a container and chilled. Some styles incorporate liqueurs such as coffee, orange and peppermint for a distinctive flavor. Chocolate mousse may be served with whipped cream and a cookie.

Gluten-Free Decision Factors:
- Ensure no flavors containing gluten
- Ensure no wheat flour as ingredient
- Request no cookie

Food Allergen Preparation Considerations:
- Contains dairy from cream, milk and possibly from chocolate and cookie
- Contains eggs as an ingredient and possibly from cookie
- May contain corn from colors or flavors in liqueurs
- May contain peanuts from cookie and various flavors
- May contain soy from colors or flavors in liqueurs and chocolate
- May contain tree nuts from cookie and various flavors

Crème Brulée (Baked Custard)

Crème Brulée is one of the most popular French

desserts and is equally popular in American Steak and Seafood restaurants. The custard is made with heavy cream, egg yolks, sugar and vanilla. The whisked ingredients are then baked. After it has cooled, it is topped with brown sugar that is caramelized by placing the custard in a broiler or torched by hand. There are many different types of *Crème Brulée,* some of which may contain different flavors such as almond, chocolate or fresh berries.

Gluten-Free Decision Factors:
- Ensure no wheat flour as ingredient

Food Allergen Preparation Considerations:
- Contains dairy from cream
- Contains eggs from egg yolks
- May contain corn from almond or vanilla extract
- May contain soy from chocolate
- May contain tree nuts from almond extract

Flourless Chocolate Torte
Yes, there is such a thing as flourless chocolate

torte…even if some pastry chefs forget the title. Butter, chocolate, eggs and sugar are the standard ingredients and ground nuts may also be added to make up for the lack of flour which would normally hold everything together. Some pastry chefs may use bread crumbs or flour, even though the title suggests they are omitted.

Gluten-Free Decision Factors:
- Ensure no wheat flour as ingredient
- Ensure no bread crumbs

Food Allergen Preparation Considerations:
- Contains dairy from butter, chocolate and possibly from bread crumbs
- Contains eggs as an ingredient and possibly from bread crumbs
- May contain corn from bread crumbs
- May contain peanuts from bread crumbs
- May contain soy from chocolate and bread crumbs
- May contain tree nuts from bread crumbs

Fresh Berries with Whipped Cream

Fresh berries in season usually include blueberries, raspberries and strawberries. Depending on your location, other types such as blackberries, boysenberries and loganberries may be available. They are served chilled and are usually topped with whipped cream.

Gluten-Free Decision Factors:
- None

Food Allergen Preparation Considerations:
- Contains dairy from whipped cream

Ice Cream

Ice cream is typically available at American Steak and Seafood restaurants. Some restaurants serve pre-fabricated ice cream, while others choose to make their own. Many ice cream brands are gluten-free and they come in big containers with clear labels. Ask your server to read the ingredients listed on the container and keep your flavor choices simple.

Gluten-Free Decision Factors:
- Ensure no flavors containing gluten

- Ensure no malt and wheat as ingredients
- Ensure no stabilizers which may contain gluten
- Request no cookie

Food Allergen Preparation Considerations:
- Contains dairy as an ingredient and possibly from chocolate and colors or flavors
- May contain corn from colors or flavors and malt
- May contain eggs from cookie
- May contain peanuts from cookie and various flavors
- May contain soy from colors or flavors, chocolate and cookie
- May contain tree nuts from cookie and various flavors

Sorbet

Sorbet is puréed fruit and sugar that is frozen and served like ice cream. Raspberry, lemon and lime sorbets are the most common, though you may encounter many other fruit flavors or chocolate. Occasionally, sorbet is served with a Pirouline, other type of cookie or wafer.

Gluten-Free Decision Factors:
- Ensure no stabilizers which may contain gluten
- Ensure no wheat as ingredient
- Request no cookie

Food Allergen Preparation Considerations:
- May contain corn from colors or flavors
- May contain dairy from chocolate, colors or flavors and cookie
- May contain eggs from cookie
- May contain peanuts from cookie and various flavors
- May contain soy from colors or flavors, chocolate and cookie
- May contain tree nuts from cookie and various flavors

American Steak and Seafood Cuisine: Quick Reference Guide
(Appetizers – Salads)

	Corn	Dairy	Eggs	Fish	Gluten/Wheat	Peanuts	Shellfish	Soy	Tree Nuts
Appetizers									
Oysters on the Half Shell	O	O	O	O	O		●	O	
Shrimp Cocktail	O		O	O	O		●	O	
Soups									
Bisque (Cream Soup)	O	●	O	O	O	O	O	O	O
Salads									
Buffalo Mozzarella and Tomato Salad	O	●			O			O	
Chopped Salad	O	O	O	O	O	O		O	
Cobb Salad	O	●	●	O	O	O		O	
Hearts of Palm Salad	O		O		O			O	
Mixed Green Salad	O	O	O	O	O	O		O	

Always ensure no cross-contamination in food preparation

● Typically contains allergen   O May contain allergen

American Steak and Seafood Cuisine: Quick Reference Guide

(Meat – Seafood Entrees)

	Corn	Dairy	Eggs	Fish	Gluten/Wheat	Peanuts	Shellfish	Soy	Tree Nuts
Meat Entrees									
Hamburgers	O	O	O		O	O		O	O
Pork Chops*	O	O			O	O		O	
Lamb Chops	O	O	O		O	O		O	O
Steaks	O	O	O		O	O		O	
Chicken Entrees									
Grilled Chicken Breast*	O	O			O	O		O	
Roasted Chicken*	O	O			O	O		O	
Seafood Entrees									
Crab	O	O	O	O	O	O	●	O	O
Fish Filet	O	O		●	O	O		O	
Lobster	O	O	O	O	O	O	●	O	O

Always ensure no cross-contamination in food preparation

● Typically contains allergen O May contain allergen

* Food allergens may vary depending upon type of accompaniment

American Steak and Seafood Cuisine: Quick Reference Guide
(Side Dishes)

Side Dishes	Corn	Dairy	Eggs	Fish	Gluten/Wheat	Peanuts	Shellfish	Soy	Tree Nuts
Asparagus	O	O	O		O	O		O	
Baked Potato	O	O			O			O	
Broccoli	O	O			O	O		O	
French Fried Potatoes	O	O			O	O		O	
Green Beans	O	O	O		O	O		O	O
Hash Browns	O	O			O	O		O	
Mashed Potatoes	O	O			O			O	
Potatoes Lyonnaise	O	O			O	O		O	
Spinach	O	O			O	O		O	

Always ensure no cross-contamination in food preparation

● Typically contains allergen O May contain allergen

American Steak and Seafood Cuisine: Quick Reference Guide
(Desserts)

Desserts	Corn	Dairy	Eggs	Fish	Gluten/Wheat	Peanuts	Shellfish	Soy	Tree Nuts
Chocolate Mousse	○	●	●		○	○		○	○
Crème Brulée (Baked Custard)	○	●	●		○			○	○
Flourless Chocolate Torte	○	●	●		○	○		○	○
Fresh Berries with Whipped Cream		●							
Ice Cream	○	●	○		○	○		○	○
Sorbet	○	○	○		○	○		○	○

Always ensure no cross-contamination in food preparation

● Typically contains allergen ○ May contain allergen

56

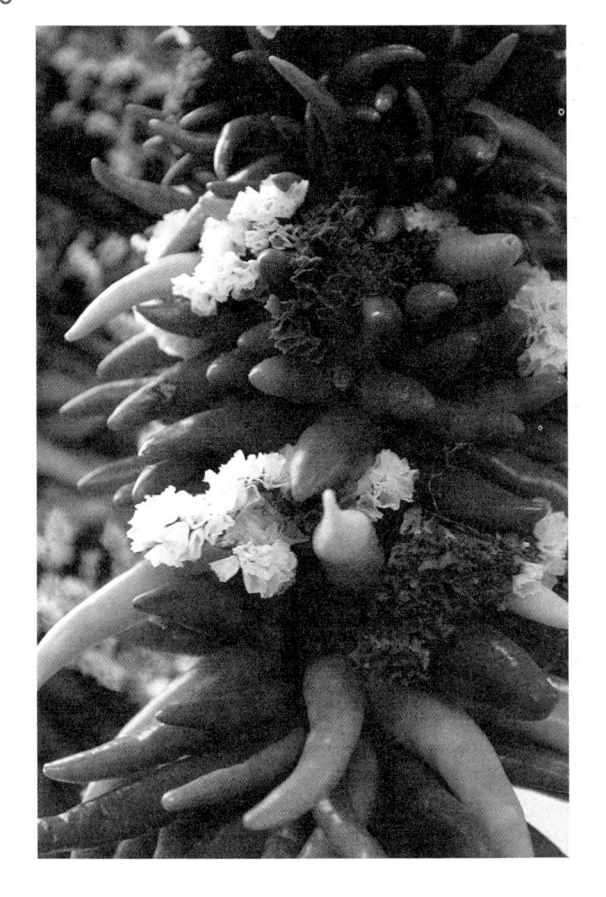

Conversation is food for the soul.
—Mexican proverb

Let's Eat Mexican Cuisine

Cuisine Overview

The following materials outline:

- Dining considerations
- Sample Mexican menu
- Mexican cuisine menu items and descriptions
- Quick reference guide

Dining Considerations

Mexican menu items are usually presented in Spanish. You may often find menu descriptions in the language of the country you are in following the name of the Mexican menu item. While traveling, be sure to familiarize yourself with the common Mexican culinary terms included in this chapter to assist you in your dining experience.

Like the Italians and French, Mexicans like to eat slowly and savor their food. The afternoon and evening meals are usually served in a modified course structure inspired by the French *service à la russe* and can last about two to three hours. This casual dining style means that the check, or *la cuenta,* is typically delivered when asked for. This relaxed style of service can often be confused with poor service. If you have time constraints, it is best to let your server know in advance so that they may expedite your meal appropriately.

Buen Provecho!

Sample Mexican Menu

Appetizers

Ceviche (Raw Fish Salad)
Chile con Queso (Chili Cheese Dip)
Guacamole (Avocado Dip)
Queso Fundido (Cheese Dip)
Tortillas y Salsa (Chips and Salsa)

Soups

Posole (Chili Corn Soup)
Sopa Azteca (Lime Chicken Soup)

Salads

Ensalada (House Salad)
Taco Salad

Egg Entrees

Huevos Mexicanos (Mexican Eggs)
Huevos Rancheros (Ranch Style Eggs)

Sample Mexican Menu

Antojos (Mexican Specialties)
Enchiladas
Enfrijoladas
Tacos
Tamales (Stuffed Corn Meal)
Tostadas Compuestas (Filled Corn Tortillas)

Meat Entrees
Arracheras (Flank or Skirt Steak)
Bistek (Steak)
Carne Asada (Broiled Beef)
Carnitas (Simmered Pork)
Machaca (Shredded Beef)

Chicken and Turkey Entrees
Mole
Pechuga de Pollo (Chicken Breast)
Pollo Asado (Broiled Chicken)

Seafood Entrees
Langosta (Lobster)
Paella Mariscos (Seafood and Rice)

Sample Mexican Menu

Side Dishes
Arroz (Rice)

Frijoles (Beans)

Desserts
Arroz con Leche (Rice Pudding)

Flan (Custard)

Helados (Ice Cream, Sherbet or Sorbet)

We would like to thank Freddie Sanchez, owner and chef of Adobo Grill in Chicago, Illinois and the Crawley Family of El Sombrero Patio Cafe in Las Cruces, New Mexico for their valuable contributions in reviewing the following menu items.

Mexican Menu Item Descriptions

Appetizers
Ceviche (Raw Fish Salad)
Ceviche is a popular appetizer enjoyed worldwide, specifically in Latin America and Spain. In most cases, it is raw white fish with chopped jalepeños, cilantro and onions tossed in lime juice with salt. Ceviche may also include other *mariscos* (seafood) such as calamari, crab, lobster, octopus or shrimp; however, these ingredients are usually cooked. The dish may be served with corn tortilla chips.

Gluten-Free Decision Factors:
- Ensure that the oil used for frying is designated for corn tortilla chips only and is not used to fry other items that may be dusted with flour

- Request corn tortilla chips—ensure no wheat flour

Food Allergen Preparation Considerations:
- Contains fish
- May contain corn from tortilla chips and vegetable oil
- May contain shellfish
- May contain peanuts from vegetable oil
- May contain soy from tortilla chips and vegetable oil

Chile con Queso (Chili Cheese Dip)

Traditional *Chile con Queso* is a blend of butter, cheese and chopped chile pepper. Any type of cheese or chile pepper can be used. It is usually served with corn tortilla chips or plain hot tortillas.

Gluten-Free Decision Factors:
- Ensure no wheat flour in sauce
- Ensure that the oil used for frying is designated for corn tortilla chips only and

is not used to fry other items that may be battered or dusted with wheat flour

- Request corn tortillas—ensure no wheat flour

Food Allergen Preparation Considerations:
- Contains dairy from butter and cheese
- May contain corn from tortilla chips and vegetable oil
- May contain peanuts from vegetable oil
- May contain soy from tortilla chips and vegetable oil

Guacamole (Avocado Dip)

Guacamole is crushed avocado with garlic, lime juice, onions and tomatoes. Other ingredients may include diced chile pepper and cilantro. It is usually served with corn tortilla chips or plain hot tortillas.

Gluten-Free Decision Factors:
- Ensure that the oil used for frying is designated for corn tortilla chips only and is not used to fry other items that may be battered or dusted with wheat flour

- Request corn tortilla chips—ensure no wheat flour

Food Allergen Preparation Considerations:
- May contain corn from tortilla chips and vegetable oil
- May contain peanuts from vegetable oil
- May contain soy from tortilla chips and vegetable oil

Queso Fundido (Cheese Dip)

Queso Fundido is another variety of Mexican cheese dip. Cheese is melted together with butter and served in a hot ceramic dish. It may include sliced vegetables such as bell peppers, onions and tomatoes. Sometimes *chorizo* (Mexican pork sausage) may be added. It is usually served with corn tortilla chips or plain hot tortillas.

Gluten-Free Decision Factors:
- Ensure no wheat flour in sauce
- Ensure oil used for frying is designated for corn tortilla chips only and is not used to fry

other items that may be battered or dusted with wheat flour

- Request corn tortillas—ensure no wheat flour

Food Allergen Preparation Considerations:
- Contains dairy from butter and cheese
- May contain corn from tortillas and vegetable oil
- May contain peanuts from vegetable oil
- May contain soy from tortillas and vegetable oil

Tortillas y Salsa (Chips and Salsa)

Any Mexican meal would be incomplete without a bowl of chips and salsa. Corn tortilla chips are accompanied by any type of fresh salsa.

Gluten-Free Decision Factors:
- Ensure no wheat flour in salsa
- Ensure that the oil used for frying is designated for corn tortilla chips only and is not used to fry other items that may be

battered or dusted with wheat flour

- Request corn tortilla chips—ensure no wheat flour

Food Allergen Preparation Considerations:
- May contain corn from salsa, tortilla chips and vegetable oil
- May contain peanuts from vegetable oil
- May contain soy from tortilla chips and vegetable oil

Soups
Posole (Chili Corn Soup)
Posole is a traditional, spicy Mexican soup. Although there are many recipes, most follow these guidelines: chunks of pork are simmered in fresh chicken stock with garlic, hominy, onions, chile peppers and tomato. With the exception of hominy, the other ingredients will likely be sautéed in oil prior to being added to the soup. It can be seasoned with *azafran* (Mexican saffron), chile powder, cilantro, Mexican oregano or any other Mexican herbs and spices. Both *Posole* and *Menudo*

(a similar soup that features tripe) are considered excellent hangover remedies in Mexico.

Gluten-Free Decision Factors:
- Ensure stocks and broths are made fresh and not from bouillon which may contain gluten
- Ensure no wheat flour as thickening agent

Food Allergen Preparation Considerations:
- Contains corn from hominy and possibly from bouillon and vegetable oil
- May contain peanuts from vegetable oil
- May contain soy from bouillon and vegetable oil

Sopa Azteca (Lime Chicken Soup)

Sopa Azteca may also be called tortilla soup on some restaurant menus. There are many variations of this soup, but most are similar in preparation. Garlic, onions, sliced chicken and tomatoes are simmered in fresh chicken stock and lime juice. The soup is often topped with crunchy corn tortilla strips and grated cheese. Some recipes call for a greater variety of vegetables and may also include cream.

Gluten-Free Decision Factors:
- Ensure no wheat flour tortillas—corn tortillas are typically used
- Ensure stocks and broths are made fresh and not from bouillon which may contain gluten
- Ensure no wheat flour as thickening agent
- Ensure oil used for frying is designated for corn tortilla chips only and is not used to fry other items that may be battered or dusted with wheat flour

Food Allergen Preparation Considerations:
- Contains dairy from cheese and possibly from cream
- May contain corn from bouillon, tortilla chips and vegetable oil
- May contain peanuts from vegetable oil
- May contain soy from bouillon, tortilla chips and vegetable oil

Salads
Ensalada (House Salad)
An *Ensalada* will usually be included with a *plato fuerte* or main dish. This salad usually consists of lettuce, onions and tomatoes. Salad dressings are uncommon; usually a wine vinegar and oil are available if needed.

Gluten-Free Decision Factors:
- None

Food Allergen Preparation Considerations:
- May contain corn from vegetable oil
- May contain peanuts from vegetable oil
- May contain soy from vegetable oil

Taco Salad
Taco salads are found on restaurant menus outside of Mexico. They can be served in a corn tortilla bowl, flour tortilla bowl or on a plate, topped with tortilla chips. The dish contains mixed greens, beans, grated cheese, onions and tomatoes. Your options usually include sliced marinated chicken,

ground beef or steak. The salad is typically topped with fresh salsa and sour cream since salad dressings are uncommon.

Gluten-Free Decision Factors:
- Ensure no soy sauce or wheat flour in marinade
- Ensure no wheat flour in salsa
- Ensure no wheat flour in beans
- Ensure oil used for frying is designated for corn tortillas only and is not used to fry other items that may be battered or dusted with wheat flour
- Request corn tortilla bowl and chips—ensure no wheat flour

Food Allergen Preparation Considerations:
- Contains dairy from cheese and sour cream
- May contain corn from salsa, tortillas and vegetable oil
- May contain peanuts from vegetable oil
- May contain soy from soy sauce in marinade, tortillas and vegetable oil

Egg Entrees
Huevos Mexicanos (Mexican Eggs)

Huevos Mexicanos are scrambled eggs with chopped chile, onions and tomatoes. Eggs are usually cooked with vegetable oil or occasionally butter. They are often served with steamed tortillas and beans, which may be topped with cheese. Salsa picante (puréed tomatoes, chile, garlic, onions and cilantro) or pico de gallo (a fresh salsa consisting of tomatoes, onions, garlic, jalapenos and cilantro) may be offered on the side.

Gluten-Free Decision Factors:
- Ensure no wheat flour in salsa
- Ensure no wheat flour in beans
- Request corn tortillas—ensure no wheat flour
- Ensure oil used for frying has not been used to fry other items which may be battered or dusted with wheat flour

Food Allergen Preparation Considerations:
- Contains eggs as ingredient
- May contain corn from salsa, tortillas and vegetable oil

- May contain dairy from butter and cheese
- May contain peanuts from vegetable oil
- May contain soy from tortillas and vegetable oil

Huevos Rancheros (Ranch Style Eggs)

Huevos Rancheros consist of eggs fried in vegetable oil or occasionally butter. They are usually sunny side up, on top of a corn tortilla that has been lightly fried in vegetable oil. The eggs are topped with chile con carne (meat simmered in red or green chile) and cheese. Chopped lettuce, onions, tomatoes, beans and pico de gallo may also accompany the dish.

Gluten-Free Decision Factors:
- Ensure no wheat flour in salsa or sauce
- Ensure no wheat flour in beans
- Ensure oil used for frying is designated for corn tortillas only and is not used to fry other items that may be battered or dusted with wheat flour

- Request corn tortillas—ensure no wheat flour

Food Allergen Preparation Considerations:
- Contains dairy from cheese and possibly from butter
- Contains eggs as ingredient
- May contain corn from salsa, tortillas and vegetable oil
- May contain peanuts from vegetable oil
- May contain soy from tortillas and vegetable oil

Antojos (Mexican Specialties)
Enchiladas

Enchiladas are prepared two different ways: rolled and stuffed with ingredients or stacked like pancakes and layered with ingredients. When rolled, the tortillas are lightly fried in vegetable oil, stuffed with the ingredients of your choice and then topped with mole, red chile sauce or green chile sauce and cheese. The stacked variety is prepared a little differently. After the tortillas have been lightly fried, they are dipped in red or green chile and then layered with the ingredients of your choice. Standard *enchilada* ingredients include cheese and onions, served plain or with your choice of beef, chicken or pork. However, there are hundreds of recipes, many of which can include any number of ingredients. Stacked *enchiladas* are often topped with a fried egg.

Gluten-Free Decision Factors:
- Ensure no wheat flour in sauce
- Ensure oil used for frying is designated for corn tortillas only and is not used to fry other items that may be battered or dusted with wheat flour
- Request corn tortillas—ensure no wheat flour

Food Allergen Preparation Considerations:
- Contains dairy from cheese and possibly from cream
- May contain corn from tortillas and vegetable oil
- May contain eggs as ingredient
- May contain peanuts from mole sauce and vegetable oil

- May contain soy from chocolate in mole sauce, tortillas and vegetable oil
- May contain tree nuts from mole sauce

Enfrijoladas

Enfrijoladas are like enchiladas, but feature beans as a major ingredient. Tortillas are lightly fried in oil then dipped in a crushed or puréed bean sauce with garlic. They can be rolled or stacked with cheese and onions and are typically topped with salsa and sour cream. Sometimes beef or chicken may be offered as fillings. Stacked *enfrijoladas* are often topped with a fried egg.

Gluten-Free Decision Factors:
- Ensure oil used for frying is designated for corn tortillas only and is not used to fry other items that may be battered or dusted with wheat flour
- Ensure no wheat flour in salsa or sauce
- Request corn tortillas—ensure no wheat flour

Food Allergen Preparation Considerations:
- Contains dairy from cheese and sour cream
- May contain corn from salsa, tortillas and vegetable oil
- May contain eggs as ingredient
- May contain peanuts from vegetable oil
- May contain soy from tortillas and vegetable oil

Tacos

Tacos are the Mexican version of a sandwich. They come in fried or steamed corn tortillas or in soft wheat flour tortillas. In most cases, they are folded; however, you may come across fried rolled tacos called *Flautas* or *Taquitos*. Ingredients vary widely depending on where you are and what type you decide to order. Some varieties include *al carbon* (grilled beef), *al dorado* (rolled and fried with shredded chicken or beef), *al pastor* (shaved marinated pork), *carnitas* (pork simmered with orange rind), *camarones* (shrimp), *machaca* (shredded beef), *pescado* (fish) and *pollo* (chicken). In addition to shredded lettuce and cheese, other garnishes may include sliced cucumbers, radishes, red and green salsas, sour cream, lime wedges and guacamole.

Gluten-Free Decision Factors:
- Ensure no wheat flour in salsa
- Ensure oil used for frying is designated for corn tortillas only and is not used to fry other items that may be battered or dusted with flour
- Request corn tortillas—ensure no wheat flour

Food Allergen Preparation Considerations:
- Contains dairy from cheese and sour cream
- May contain corn from salsa, tortillas and vegetable oil
- May contain fish if ordered
- May contain shellfish if ordered
- May contain peanuts from vegetable oil
- May contain soy from tortillas and vegetable oil

Tamales (Stuffed Corn Meal)

Tamales are made of *masa* (corn meal and vegetable oil or lard), which is stuffed with various ingredients, wrapped in a corn husk and steamed. There are a number of different types of tamale ingredients, the most common being shredded beef, chicken or pork that is simmered in red chile sauce.

Gluten-Free Decision Factors:
- Ensure no wheat flour in sauce

Food Allergen Preparation Considerations:
- Contains corn from *masa* and possibly from vegetable oil

- May contain peanuts from vegetable oil

- May contain soy from *masa* and from vegetable oil

Tostadas Compuestas (Filled Corn Tortillas)

Tostadas Compuestas are crisp fried corn tortillas, either flat or shaped in a bowl, which are topped or filled with various ingredients. The most common are red or green chile con carne, shredded cheese, lettuce and tomatoes. Some recipes may also call for beans, sliced marinated beef or chicken, pico de gallo and sour cream.

Gluten-Free Decision Factors:
- Ensure no wheat flour in salsa
- Ensure no wheat flour in beans
- Ensure no soy sauce or wheat flour in marinade
- Ensure oil used for frying is designated for corn tortillas only and is not used to fry other items that may be battered or dusted with wheat flour
- Request corn tortillas—ensure no wheat flour

Food Allergen Preparation Considerations:
- Contains dairy from cheese and possibly sour cream
- May contain corn from salsa, tortillas and vegetable oil
- May contain peanuts from vegetable oil
- May contain soy from soy sauce in marinade, tortillas and vegetable oil

Meat Entrees
Arracheras (Flank or Skirt Steak)

Arracheras are thin cuts of meat and are used for making fajitas. The only real difference between the two is that fajitas are sliced into thinner strips. Flank or skirt steak is marinated in lime juice, garlic, salt, pepper and sometimes diced chile peppers. The beef is cooked over an open flame to temperature and served with steamed tortillas, shredded lettuce, tomatoes, beans and rice. The beans may be topped with cheese and salsa picante or pico de gallo.

Gluten-Free Decision Factors:
- Ensure no wheat flour in salsa
- Ensure no wheat flour in beans
- Ensure no soy sauce or wheat flour in marinade
- Request corn tortillas—ensure no wheat flour

Food Allergen Preparation Considerations:
- May contain corn from salsa, tortillas and vegetable oil in beans
- May contain dairy from cheese

- May contain peanuts from vegetable oil in beans

- May contain soy from soy sauce in marinade, tortillas and vegetable oil in beans

Bistek (Steak)

Steaks come in a variety of cuts, the most popular being filet, New York strip, porterhouse, and rib eye. The type of cut varies widely depending upon where you are eating and what is available at any given restaurant. Steaks are generally seasoned with salt and pepper and broiled or grilled. They may also be marinated in fresh lime juice, garlic and diced chile peppers. Beans (which may be topped with cheese) and rice are common side dishes. You may also encounter *papas fritas* (fried potatoes). Occasionally a menu will offer *Bistek Ranchero*, in which case the beef is smothered in salsa ranchero.

Gluten-Free Decision Factors:
- Ensure no wheat flour in salsa

- Ensure no wheat flour in beans

- Ensure no soy sauce or wheat flour in marinade
- Ensure oil used for frying is designated for potatoes only and is not used to fry other items that may be battered or dusted with wheat flour

Food Allergen Preparation Considerations:
- May contain corn from salsa, vegetable oil in beans and fried potatoes
- May contain dairy from cheese
- May contain peanuts from vegetable oil in beans
- May contain soy from soy sauce in marinade and vegetable oil in beans and fried potatoes

Carne Asada (Broiled Beef)

Carne Asada is marinated broiled beef and can be any of the smaller cuts of beef not considered bistek. These types include everything from butt steak to tri-tip. Mexican restaurants generally season *Carne Asada* with a marinade of lime juice, garlic, Mexican oregano, salt, pepper, and sometimes diced chile peppers. The dish is usually served with steamed tortillas, shredded lettuce, tomatoes, rice and beans, which may be topped with cheese. Salsa picante or pico de gallo may be offered on the side.

Gluten-Free Decision Factors:
- Ensure no wheat flour in salsa
- Ensure no wheat flour in beans
- Ensure no soy sauce or wheat flour in marinade
- Request corn tortillas—ensure no wheat flour

Food Allergen Preparation Considerations:
- May contain corn from salsa, tortillas and vegetable oil in beans
- May contain dairy from cheese
- May contain peanuts from vegetable oil
- May contain soy from soy sauce in marinade, tortillas and vegetable oil in beans

Carnitas (Simmered Pork)

Carnitas are a popular delicacy all over Mexico. Pork is slowly roasted and simmered in its own juices with orange rinds and any number of Mexican spices. In fact, purveyors of *Carnitas* in Mexico closely guard the specific spices they use; however, these secret recipes typically consist of dried Mexican chile powders and herbs such as cumin, *epazote* (wormseed), garlic, Mexican oregano, salt and pepper. The dish is usually served with steamed tortillas, shredded lettuce, tomatoes, rice and beans, which may be topped with cheese. Salsa picante or pico de gallo may be offered on the side.

Gluten-Free Decision Factors:
- Ensure no wheat flour in salsa
- Ensure no wheat flour in beans
- Request corn tortillas—ensure no wheat flour

Food Allergen Preparation Considerations:
- May contain corn from salsa, tortillas and vegetable oil in beans
- May contain dairy from cheese

- May contain peanuts from vegetable oil in beans
- May contain soy from tortillas and vegetable oil in beans

Machaca (Shredded Beef)

Machaca is a Northern Mexican specialty. Beef shoulder or chuck roast is simmered for hours in water, oil and spices (usually chile powder, cumin, garlic, salt and pepper). Once all the fat has been cooked out of the beef, it is pulled apart or shredded. The dish is usually served with steamed tortillas, shredded lettuce, tomatoes, rice and beans, which may be topped with cheese. Salsa picante or pico de gallo may be offered on the side.

Gluten-Free Decision Factors:
- Ensure no wheat flour in salsa
- Ensure no wheat flour in beans
- Request corn tortillas—ensure no wheat flour

Food Allergen Preparation Considerations:
- May contain corn from salsa, tortillas and vegetable oil

- May contain dairy from cheese
- May contain peanuts from vegetable oil
- May contain soy from tortillas and vegetable oil

Chicken and Turkey Entrees
Mole
Mole is a specialty from the states of Puebla and Oaxaca. It is a thick brown sauce, usually served over chicken or turkey. Although there are hundreds, if not thousands, of recipes for *Mole*, the sauce is typically made from a lengthy list of ingredients that include unsweetened chocolate, chile peppers, cinnamon, cloves, coriander, cumin, garlic, peanuts, sesame seeds, and tree nuts. The dish is usually served with steamed tortillas, shredded lettuce, tomatoes, rice and beans, which may be topped with cheese. Salsa picante or pico de gallo may be offered on the side.

Gluten-Free Decision Factors:
- Ensure no wheat flour in sauce
- Ensure no wheat flour in beans

- Request corn tortillas—ensure no wheat flour

Food Allergen Preparation Considerations:
- May contain corn from tortillas and vegetable oil in beans
- May contain dairy from cheese
- May contain peanuts from sauce and vegetable oil in beans
- May contain soy from chocolate, tortillas and vegetable oil in beans
- May contain tree nuts from sauce

Pechuga de Pollo (Chicken Breast)

Chicken breasts are usually marinated in lime juice, garlic, Mexican oregano, salt, pepper and sometimes diced chile peppers. They are cooked *asado* (broiled) or *a la parilla* (grilled). The dish is usually served with steamed tortillas, shredded lettuce, tomatoes, rice and beans, which may be topped with cheese. Salsa picante or pico de gallo may be offered on the side.

Gluten-Free Decision Factors:
- Ensure no wheat flour in salsa
- Ensure no wheat flour in beans
- Ensure no soy sauce or wheat flour in marinade
- Request corn tortillas—ensure no wheat flour

Food Allergen Preparation Considerations:
- May contain corn from salsa, tortillas and vegetable oil in beans
- May contain dairy from cheese
- May contain peanuts from vegetable oil in beans
- May contain soy from soy sauce in marinade, tortillas and vegetable oil in beans

Pollo Asado (Broiled Chicken)

Pollo Asado is a whole chicken, usually marinated in lime juice, garlic, Mexican oregano, salt, pepper and sometimes diced chile peppers. It is then broiled or charbroiled so that the skin is very crispy. The standard serving is half of a chicken on the bone. The dish is usually served with steamed tortillas, shredded lettuce, tomatoes, rice and beans, which may be topped with cheese. Salsa picante or pico de gallo may be offered on the side.

Gluten-Free Decision Factors:
- Ensure no wheat flour in salsa
- Ensure no wheat flour in beans
- Ensure no soy sauce or wheat flour in marinade
- Request corn tortillas—ensure no wheat flour

Food Allergen Preparation Considerations:
- May contain corn from salsa, tortillas and vegetable oil in beans
- May contain dairy from cheese
- May contain peanuts from vegetable oil in beans
- May contain soy from soy sauce in marinade, tortillas and vegetable oil in beans

Seafood Entrees
Langosta (Lobster)
Mexican restaurants generally offer the clawless spiny lobsters available in the Caribbean or off the coast of the Baja peninsula. Whole lobster or just the tails may be featured on the menu. Lobster tails are usually broiled or grilled, whereas whole lobsters are traditionally boiled in water, fish stock or seafood stock. Most lobster is served with drawn butter (melted butter and vegetable oil), lime wedges and steamed tortillas. Salsa picante or pico de gallo may be offered on the side.

Gluten-Free Decision Factors:
- Ensure no wheat flour in salsa
- Ensure stocks and broths are made fresh and not from bouillon which may contain gluten
- Request corn tortillas—ensure no wheat flour

Food Allergen Preparation Considerations:
- Contains shellfish from lobster and possibly from seafood stock
- May contain corn from bouillon, salsa, tortillas and vegetable oil in drawn butter

- May contain dairy from drawn butter
- May contain fish from seafood stock
- May contain peanuts from vegetable oil in drawn butter
- May contain soy from bouillon, tortillas and vegetable oil in drawn butter

Paella Mariscos (Seafood and Rice)

Paella is a popular Spanish rice dish that is enjoyed all over the Latin world including Mexican restaurants. Rice is boiled in fresh chicken or fish stock. Clams, calamari, fish, mussels, scallops and shrimp that have been sautéed in vegetable oil, herbs and spices are then added. These herbs and spices usually include *azafran* (Mexican saffron), chile powder, garlic, salt and pepper. The dish usually includes bell peppers, sliced chile peppers, onions and tomatoes.

Gluten-Free Decision Factors:
- Ensure stocks and broths are made fresh and not from bouillon which may contain gluten

Food Allergen Preparation Considerations:
- Contains fish
- Contains shellfish
- May contain corn from bouillon and vegetable oil
- May contain peanuts from vegetable oil
- May contain soy from bouillon and vegetable oil

Side Dishes
Arroz (Rice)
Most rice served in Mexican restaurants is similar in preparation and may be referred to as Spanish rice. After the rice has been boiled, usually in water or fresh chicken stock, crushed tomatoes or tomato sauce and sliced onions are added. Sometimes the tomatoes and onions may be sautéed in vegetable oil prior to being added. The rice is seasoned with salt and may also be seasoned with *azafran*.

Gluten-Free Decision Factors:
- Ensure stocks and broths are made fresh and not from bouillon which may contain gluten

Food Allergen Preparation Considerations:
- May contain corn from bouillon and vegetable oil
- May contain peanuts from vegetable oil
- May contain soy from bouillon and vegetable oil

Frijoles (Beans)

Pinto beans are the most popular variety in Northern Mexico, while black beans are mostly enjoyed in southern Mexico. Dried beans are boiled until soft, then mashed and fried with lard or oil to make *Frijoles*. This preparation style is called *Frijoles Refritos* or "refried beans" and is typically topped with cheese. Beans can also be served whole in their own broth and may be flavored with salted pork.

Gluten-Free Decision Factors:
- Ensure no wheat flour in beans

Food Allergen Preparation Considerations:
- May contain corn from vegetable oil
- May contain dairy from cheese

- May contain peanuts from vegetable oil
- May contain soy from vegetable oil

Desserts
Arroz con Leche (Rice Pudding)
Mexican rice pudding is a great dessert choice. Rice is boiled with cinnamon until soft. Milk or cream, raisins, sugar and vanilla beans or extract are then added. This is heated for a few minutes, then eggs and more cinnamon are added. This dessert can be served chilled or warm.

Gluten-Free Decision Factors:
- None

Food Allergen Preparation Considerations:
- Contains dairy from milk or cream
- Contains eggs as ingredient
- May contain corn from vanilla extract

Flan (Custard)

Flan is the national dessert of Spain and it is a common dessert in most Latin cuisines. Its ingredients are simple: cream, eggs, sugar and vanilla beans or extract. You may see it on the menu as *"Flan con Dulce de Leche,"* which means it is topped with caramel sauce.

Gluten-Free Decision Factors:
- Ensure no wheat flour

Food Allergen Preparation Considerations:
- Contains dairy from cream
- Contains eggs as ingredient
- May contain corn from caramel sauce and vanilla extract

Helados (Ice Cream, Sherbet or Sorbet)

Helados are usually available in Mexican restaurants. Many establishments make these items in-house, yet others prefer to offer pre-fabricated *Helados*. It is generally best to keep your flavor choices simple. In either case, inquire about the ingredients.

Gluten-Free Decision Factors:
- Ensure no malt or wheat as ingredients
- Ensure no stabilizers which may contain gluten
- Request no cookie

Food Allergen Preparation Considerations:
- May contain corn from caramel, colors or flavors
- May contain dairy as ingredient, from cookie and possibly from chocolate
- May contain eggs from cookie
- May contain peanuts from various flavors and from cookie
- May contain soy from chocolate, colors or flavors
- May contain tree nuts from cookie and various flavors

Mexican Cuisine: Quick Reference Guide
(Appetizers – Salads)

	Corn	Dairy	Eggs	Fish	Gluten/Wheat	Peanuts	Shellfish	Soy	Tree Nuts
Appetizers									
Ceviche (Raw Fish Salad)	O			●	O	O	O	O	
Chile con Queso (Chili Cheese Dip)	O	●			O	O		O	
Guacamole (Avocado Dip)	O				O	O		O	
Queso Fundido (Cheese Dip)	O	●			O	O		O	
Tortillas y Salsa (Chips and Salsa)	O				O	O		O	
Soups									
Posole (Chili Corn Soup)	●				O	O		O	
Sopa Azteca (Lime Chicken Soup)	O	●			O	O		O	
Salads									
Ensalada (House Salad)	O					O		O	
Taco Salad	O	●			O	O		O	

Always ensure no cross-contamination in food preparation

● Typically contains allergen   O May contain allergen

Mexican Cuisine: Quick Reference Guide
(Egg Entrees – Antojos)

	Corn	Dairy	Eggs	Fish	Gluten/Wheat	Peanuts	Shellfish	Soy	Tree Nuts
Egg Entrees									
Huevos Mexicanos (Mexican Eggs)	○	○	●		○	○		○	
Huevos Rancheros (Ranch Style Eggs)	○	●	●		○	○		○	
Antojos (Mexican Specialties)									
Enchiladas	○	●	○		○	○		○	○
Enfrijoladas	○	●	○		○	○		○	
Tacos	○	●		○	○	○	○	○	
Tamales (Stuffed Corn Meal)	●				○	○		○	
Tostadas Compuestas (Filled Corn Tortillas)	○	●			○	○		○	

Always ensure no cross-contamination in food preparation
● Typically contains allergen ○ May contain allergen

Mexican Cuisine: Quick Reference Guide
(Meat, Chicken and Turkey Entrees)

	Corn	Dairy	Eggs	Fish	Gluten/Wheat	Peanuts	Shellfish	Soy	Tree Nuts
Meat Entrees									
Arracheras (Flank or Skirt Steak)	O	O			O	O		O	
Bistek (Steak)	O	O			O	O		O	
Carne Asada (Broiled Beef)	O	O			O	O		O	
Carnitas (Simmered Pork)	O	O			O	O		O	
Machaca (Shredded Beef)	O	O			O	O		O	
Chicken and Turkey Entrees									
Mole	O	O			O	O		O	O
Pechuga de Pollo (Chicken Breast)	O	O			O	O		O	
Pollo Asado (Broiled Chicken)	O	O			O	O		O	

Always ensure no cross-contamination in food preparation
- ● Typically contains allergen
- O May contain allergen

Mexican Cuisine: Quick Reference Guide
(Seafood Entrees – Desserts)

	Corn	Dairy	Eggs	Fish	Gluten/Wheat	Peanuts	Shellfish	Soy	Tree Nuts
Seafood Entrees									
Langosta (Lobster)	O	O		O	O	O	●	O	
Paella Mariscos (Seafood and Rice)	O			●	O	O	●	O	
Side Dishes									
Arroz (Rice)	O				O	O		O	
Frijoles (Beans)	O	O			O	O		O	
Desserts									
Arroz con Leche (Rice Pudding)	O	●	●						
Flan (Custard)	O	●	●		O				
Helados (Ice Cream, Sherbet or Sorbet)	O	O	O		O	O		O	O

Always ensure no cross-contamination in food preparation

● Typically contains allergen   O May contain allergen

About the Authors and Additional Products

The following information highlights:

- Background of authors
- Additional books and passports

Background of Authors

Kim Koeller has spent the last 23 years eating 80% of her meals in restaurants across the globe while managing over a dozen food-related allergies/sensitivities and celiac/coeliac disease. Robert La France has spent over twelve years in